Pathway to ICU

Pathway to ICU

Your constant companion during a transition to ICU nursing.

Karen Ann Thompson M.S., RN

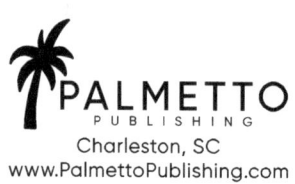

Pathway to ICU

Copyright © 2023 by Karen Ann Thompson M.S., RN

All rights reserved

No portion of this book may be reproduced, stored in a retrieval system, or transmitted in any form by any means–electronic, mechanical, photocopy, recording, or other–except for brief quotations in printed reviews, without prior permission of the author.

First Edition

Paperback ISBN: 979-8-8229-2007-1
Hardcover ISBN: 979-8-8229-3719-2

Table of Contents

Introduction 1
Certifications 3
Communication 4
Critical Thinking 6
Compassion 8
Death and Dying 9
Advocacy. 12
Resources and References 13
Resources 33
Notes 37

Introduction

Welcome to the beginning of your journey as you transition into the ICU. The purpose of this handbook is to offer various suggestions and information that will aid your transfer from being a floor nurse to an ICU nurse as well as offer resources that you can return to in the future. You'll also familiarize yourself with some of the knowledge and skills expected of an ICU nurse, learn the value of critical thinking and compassion, and review potential scenarios you might encounter.

While there is no one mold for an ICU nurse, there are abilities and positive mindsets that can set you up for success. ICU nurses are analytical and fast learners, something you must be in order to retain new information and brainstorm methods of treatment. Effective communication is vital, whether that means communicating with patients, families, fellow nurses, or doctors. We hope to see empathetic nurses who are quick to respond when a need arises!

It's important to go into any new position with the proper expectations, and this is especially true for those transferring from the floor to the ICU. By managing your expectations now, you'll pave the way for a much smoother transition. Here are some tips to keep in mind before you transfer to the ICU:

- Know that you're likely going to be overwhelmed at first. Preparing for this might be difficult, but being aware of it can help with managing stress.
- Don't be afraid to ask for help from mentors and staff or to take notes until you get the hang of things.
- Familiarize yourself with the equipment you'll be using. Before joining the ICU, also familiarize yourself with the medicines you can be expected to administer.
- Communicate with a manager related to your skill set. Try taking on some shadow shifts in the ICU in addition to your floor nurse position.
- Be prepared to deal with a different number of patients than you're used to. Mainly there will be fewer patients, but their conditions will be more complex.
- ICU is intense due to patients suffering from serious injuries or illnesses, and as a result, it requires more intense patient assessment. This can test your ability to multitask and complete tasks in a timely manner.

- Any career change is a period of transition. Recognize that what one person might excel at another may find difficult. Yet, your health care system will be dedicated to aiding you in your growth and success when it comes to transferring to the ICU and be excited for you to begin this self-directed journey!

To be successful in the ICU, "you need to build very strong fundamentals to include critical thinking and skill sets."

—Agi, veteran ICU nurse

"Be prepared for an intense and fast-paced environment with acute patients. You need to adapt to any situation with no personal biases. As far as communication is concerned, the nurse is the bridge between the MD and patient."

—Debra, charge nurse, medical ICU

Videos to Watch

- *Tips for Transitioning from Med/Surg to ICU!!*: TIPS FOR TRANSITIONING FROM MED/SURG TO ICU!! https://www.youtube.com/watch?v=DsYH8uy4nPI&feature=youtu.be

- *Must-know Tips for the New ICU Nurse*: https://www.youtube.com/watch?v=WY3rNbUEvXI

Certifications

Once you've decided to pursue a career in the ICU, you'll want to make sure you either already have or are in the process of earning your necessary certifications. This will enable you to perform not only more swiftly but also with greater confidence. As you progress through the ICU, you can get further certifications essential to critical-care nursing. These include but are not limited to:

- Basic Life Support (BLS)
- Advanced Cardiac Life Support (ACLS)
- Basic arrhythmia
- EKG interpretation
- CCRN

Just as important as earning these certifications is keeping them active; renewing any licenses that have run out will ensure you're up to date and able to carry out duties in the ICU. Along with your licenses and certifications, you'll need to be familiar with vent settings, dosages, drip medicines, and hemodynamics to be an efficient nurse.

Videos to Watch

- *Ventilator Basics for ICU I*: https://www.youtube.com/watch?v=SgTjYZD5SYE&list=PLno-hGHlBer6_KqqUpF1FkKNA_BnTzw-s&index=3

- *Ventilator Basics for ICU II*: https://www.youtube.com/watch?v=qlVAk7WSTHI&list=PLno-hGHlBer6_KqqUpF1FkKNA_BnTzw-s&index=1

- *Sedation in ICU*: https://www.youtube.com/watch?v=KF7WhB5OvCQ&list=PLno-hGHlBer6_KqqUpF1FkKNA_BnTzw-s&index=5

Communication

Nursing and effective communication are inseparable; to succeed as a critical care nurse, you must interact with people of different ethnicities, beliefs, and socioeconomic backgrounds. From patients and their families to coworkers and security, nurses are in constant communication with others. Although the ICU moves at a quicker pace than other nursing environments, taking the time to engage with patients and their families can benefit the overall well-being of those you're caring for. Showing empathy when interacting with patients reminds them that you're invested in their healing.

Engaging with overseeing doctors as well as the employees you might encounter from different floors is just as important; your ability to convey information accurately to the medical provider will affect how a patient's treatment plan is created. Communication is not just speaking; it's also documentation. Keeping up with when and which medicines are administered, when wounds have been re-dressed, and even your process for completing a task will set the groundwork for successful work relations.

Communication skills differ from person to person, and we convey information in various ways. Active listening, observation, and one's ability to present information in a straightforward manner all play a role in communication. By being aware of how you want to be communicated with and the ways you communicate with others, you will ensure a smooth transition to the ICU.

Videos to Watch

- *Communication in the ICU*: https://www.youtube.com/watch?v=GVu_sDBKtt0

- *Communication and Teamwork in the ICU*: https://www.youtube.com/watch?v=iT_gbSjLbwY "Figure 1: Passive Interaction & Superficial Relationship."

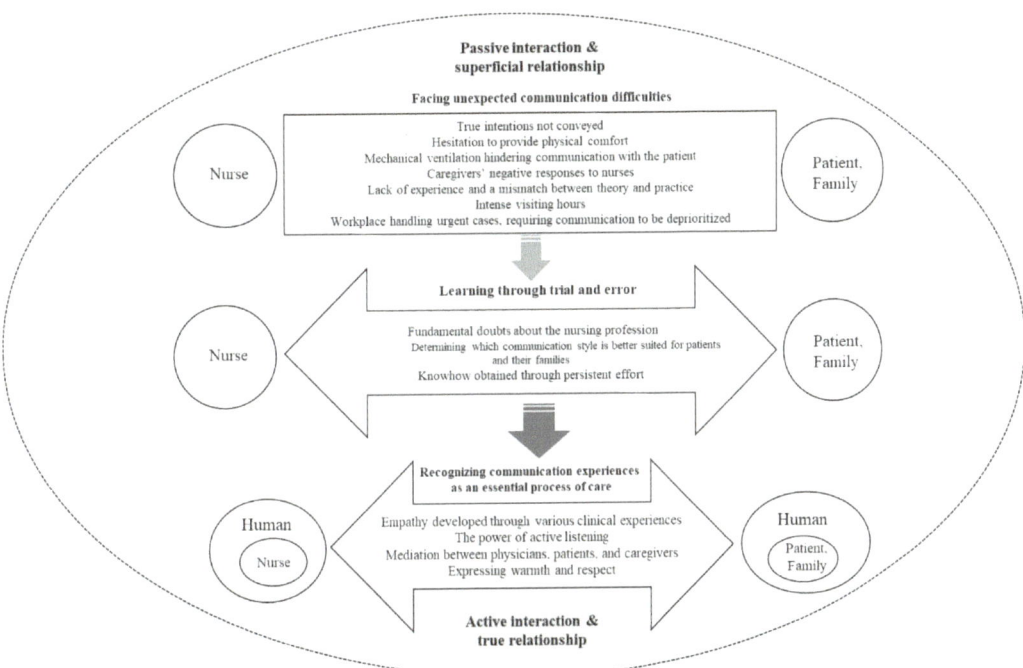

Reproduced with permission from Hai Jin Yoo et al., "Critical Care Nurses' Communication Experiences with Patients and Families in an Intensive Care Unit: A Qualitative Study." *PLOS ONE*, 15 (7). https://doi.org/10.1371/journal.pone.0235694

Critical Thinking

Working in the ICU means thinking on your feet. When issues arise, it's up to you to problem solve before calling the MD. Once you do page the doctor, already having a potential solution can save time and resources and improve the patient's quality of care. For example, imagine you're faced with a patient who's hypotensive on vasopressors, and their blood pressure decreases. What would you do if the cause is not obvious? Some questions to think about critically are:

- What is going on?
- What information am I missing?
- Can I get that information?
- What does that information mean for the patient?
- How quickly should I act? (Morris, 2023)

For those who haven't practiced critical thinking in their work, using a process may help develop these skills. Try to do the following:

1. Identify a problem or issue.
2. Create inferences about why the problem exists and how it can be solved.
3. Collect information or data on the issue through research.
4. Organize and sort data and findings.
5. Develop and execute solutions.
6. Analyze which solutions worked or didn't work.
7. Identify ways to improve the solution (Harris, 2023).

Reviewing the medicines that have been administered and lab results can sometimes offer explanations as to what may be causing the issue. If the solution still isn't clear, try brainstorming with a fellow nurse or supervisor to consider different treatment options. When you do call for the doctor, clearly conveying the issue—both to them and the patient—will allow for a more straightforward and accurate assessment.

To succeed both as a nurse and a critical thinker, you need to think beyond the tasks you're assigned. While you might be charged with changing a patient's wound dressing or monitoring vitals, these are NOT the only things you're expected to do. Critically thinking about future tasks can help with potential dilemmas, such as a medication causing a patient's blood pressure to drop. Add in the fact that you'll be managing multiple patients and mentally keeping their treatments and conditions separate to ensure their safety, and critical thinking becomes an even more important skill to develop.

Videos to Watch

- *Critical Thinking Exercises for Nurses at the Time of Emergency*: https://www.youtube.com/watch?v=5TR_2GYPOdY

- *How to Improve Critical Thinking Skills*: https://www.youtube.com/watch?v=NCf2IvEGUOU

Compassion

At the heart of every great nurse is compassion. Being compassionate in your everyday life will carry over into your work life. No matter your experience, all nurses must show a readiness to empathize with their patients and make sure the care they offer reflects this. Compassionate nursing reminds patients and their loved ones that they matter. A kind word and a caring disposition can bring comfort and improve patient outcomes dramatically. But being compassionate doesn't stop with patients; showing kindness to your peers and supervisors can eliminate some of the stress that comes with working in the ICU. Ultimately, compassion paves the way for better working relationships.

Four Skills Needed to Deliver Compassionate Care

1. Emotional Intelligence. Having an awareness of your emotions as well as the emotions of others means you can empathize with people and deliver more compassionate care.
2. Confidence. Being confident in your abilities allows you to better craft an environment where nurse-patient relations and patient outcomes are positive.
3. Cultural Awareness. Appreciating the diverse cultures within patient populations will aid you as you engage with people who have different beliefs and perspectives.
4. Patience. Taking the time to get to know patients and showing an interest in them will remind them they are not simply another task to be checked off a list, but people with specific needs and interests. (Faubion, n.d.)

Compassion is the essence of nursing. All nurses must exhibit some level of compassion to be accomplished both professionally and personally and so that they may improve patient outcomes.

Videos to Watch

- *Compassionate Care in the ICU Professional Version*: https://www.youtube.com/watch?v=t9Ic_Rkdbi4

- *Compassion, Dignity and Respect in Health Care*: https://www.youtube.com/watch?v=HVF0273iHus

Death and Dying

Death and dying can and does happen in the hospital, especially in the ICU. Whatever experience you have with losing a patient or the procedures to be considered when administering requested care and notifying family, nurses must adhere to the patient's wishes if applicable and work together to ensure there isn't a lack of communication between doctors and the patient and their family.

Adjusting your expectations of death and dying may be beneficial as you join the ICU. Often, nurses coming from a floor position have little to no experience with dying patients and may be overwhelmed by how unexpected or prologued death in the ICU can be. Try to reflect on your perception of death, as painful as it may be visualizing how you'd wish to be treated if you were dying or had a loved one dying can help you prepare for such a situation. Drawing on experiences of comforting a dying family member or patient in your nursing tenure can also help.

You'll need to think about approaches for treating terminal patients as well. Have they signed a DNR order or refused intubation despite being in respiratory failure? Does the family indicate that they want their loved one to be resuscitated? Knowing these answers prior to performing any treatment or lifesaving action can guarantee the patient's wishes are met and that they receive the dignity they deserve. To ensure a patient passes with dignity though, you must make sure communication channels are clear and that you're readily sharing information with nurses and doctors.

Scenario 48 from the TeamSTEPPS® Instructor Manual: Specialty Scenarios

"A forty-four-year-old female is admitted to the medical ICU in acute respiratory distress with upper and lower GI bleeding. Her past medical history is significant for end-stage liver disease due to alcohol abuse. The patient is intubated in response to worsening respiratory distress, aggressively resuscitated, and given blood transfusion and vasopressor drugs. Multiple consultation services are involved in the patient's care. All recommend that the patient's DNR status be addressed. Eight hours into her stay, a member of the GI consultation team places a call to the patient's mother, who lives out of state. Her mother is aware that her daughter has end-stage liver disease and states that her daughter would not want all these things done, and they should be stopped. Over the next six hours, however, the patient continues to be aggressively resuscitated. At sixteen hours into her stay, the patient's blood pressure begins to drop. The MICU physician comes to the patient's bedside and pronounces her dead.

Approximately twenty hours after the patient's arrival, the patient's mother calls to ask about her condition. She is very upset at failing to be notified of her daughter's death four hours earlier.

Instructor Comments: In this scenario, a shared mental model and advocate is lacking. When new information is obtained by a team member, it should be called out to the team by a formal handoff. No leader or team actions are taken to identify and determine the patient's DNR status. Upon that determination, the team briefs, or huddles regarding the appropriate plan of care, and everyone has a shared mental model.

Skills Needed: Team structure, mutual support, and a shared mental model.

Potential Tools: A brief, huddle, handoff, and collaboration." (Team Stepps instructor manual, 2022)

A patient may pass swiftly, or their death may be lengthy; no matter the case, how you approach this and best help their loved one's cope requires empathy. Remembering that no death will be the same will also influence how you go about interacting with family members. For instance, if a patient's family is not religious, would you recommend they visit the chaplain? How would you speak to a patient who refuses a necessary blood transfusion because it's against their beliefs? There is no single way to anticipate what can happen in any given situation, but being adaptable to your patient's needs and requests—and those of their loved ones—shows commitment.

Self-Reflection Activity

Scenario #1: You have a patient suffering from acute coronary syndrome who is likely not to survive. How would you respond if the patient doesn't accept their diagnosis and becomes agitated? How would you approach the family? In what ways can you buffer a doctor's diagnosis if it comes across too harshly? Would you recommend supportive medicine to ease the patient's pain?

Scenario #2: A patient who was recovering well from a gunshot wound dies suddenly, and the family is in shock. How would you show them compassion? Do you offer to sit with them in silence or to bring them a drink? What steps would you take to make sure all the information they request regarding treatment (or lack of treatment) is accurate?

Videos to Watch

- *Nurses on Death and Dying*: https://www.youtube.com/watch?v=j_FR-JVpnx8

- *How Doctors Tell Patients They're Dying | Being Mortal | FRONTLINE*: https://www.youtube.com/watch?v=jaB9M8B_Tuw

Advocacy

Showing support for your place of work may not always be at the forefront of your mind, but nurses who advocate for their department become part of that hospital's culture and set an example for others. More important than this though is that nurses can often put change in motion by advocating for their patients. This includes serving as intermediary between patients and their doctors; making sure patients retain as much autonomy as possible; protecting the rights, beliefs, and safety of patients by acting on their behalf; and even being vocal in the community about adequate nursing standards and health care.

Ways to Advocate as a Nurse

1. Mediate conversations between patients and physicians.
2. When needed, suggest resources to patients related to treatment or involving financial assistance.
3. Educate your patients.
4. Continue to educate yourself.
5. Advocate for legal choices or policy changes.
6. Advocate for and care for yourself (Indeed, 2022a).

Being a successful nurse advocate will call on your ability to communicate with others, your critical thinking skills, and your willingness to empathize with people no matter the situation.

Videos to Watch

- *The Important Role of Nurse Patient Advocates*: https://www.youtube.com/watch?v=ndAM8h7ASHs

- *Nurses Defined: Patient Advocacy*: https://www.youtube.com/watch?v=BNdIsc2zQLk

Resources and References

Charts and Tables

DISCLAIMER

Always consult and follow your facility's policy and guidelines. The information in this file is not to be used in substitution of your institution's policies, procedures, or guidelines. This file is a supplementary resource only.

Written permission given to use these images from Thenursefilesco @ Etsy. Additional images available for download.

For more resources, please see Thenursefilesco on Etsy.com and nursewisedownloads.etsy.com.

These files are for the sole purchaser only and may not be resold, copied, distributed, altered, shared, or used for commercial use. All information provided in this file may only be used for personal purposes and is never to be shared with others online or in person.

EKG INTERPRETATION RESOURCE

Arrhythmias	Description	Causes	Treatment
Paroxysmal Supraventricular Tachycardia 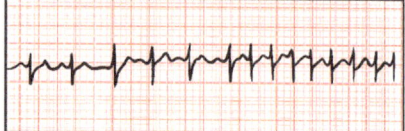	• Atrial and ventricular rhythms are regular. • Heart rate > 160 bpm rarely exceeds 250 bpm. • P wave regular but aberrant; difficult to differentiate from preceding T waves. • P wave preceding each QRS complex. • Sudden onset and termination of arrhythmia. • When a normal P wave is present, it's called paroxysmal atrial tachycardia; when a normal P wave isn't present, it's called paroxysmal junctional tachycardia.	• Physical exertion, emotion, stimulants, rheumatic heart diseases. • Intrinsic abnormality of AV conduction system. • Digoxin toxicity. • Use of caffeine, marijuana or central nervous system stimulants.	• If the patient is unstable prepare for immediate cardioversion. • If the patient is stable, vagal stimulation or Valsalva's maneuver, carotid sinus massage. • Adenosine by rapid LV bolus injection to rapidly convert arrhythmia. • If a patient has normal ejection fraction, consider a calcium channel blockers, beta-adrenergic blocks or amiodarone. • If a patient has an ejection fraction less than 40% consider amiodarone.

Description	Causes	Treatment	Arrhythmias
• Atrial rhythm regular, rate 250 to 400 bpm. • Ventricular rate variable, depending on degree of AV block. • Saw-tooth shape P wave configuration. • QRS complexes are uniform in shape but often irregular in rate.	• Heart failure, tricuspid or mitral valve disease, pulmonary embolism, cor pulmonale, inferior wall MI, carditis. • Digoxin toxicity	• If a patient is unstable with ventricular rate >150 bpm, prepare for immediate cardioversion. • If the patient is stable, drug therapy may include calcium channel blockers, beta adrenergic block, or antiarrhythmic. • Anticoagulation therapy may be necessary.	**Atrial Flutter** 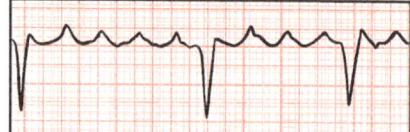

Arrhythmias	Description	Causes	Treatment
Atrial Fibrillation 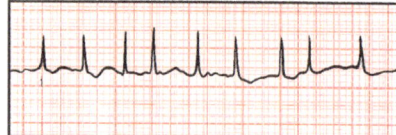	• Atrial rhythm grossly irregular rate > 300 to 600 bpm. • Ventricular rhythm grossly irregular, rate 160 to 180 bpm. • PR interval indiscernible. • No P waves, or P waves that appear as erratic, irregular base-line fibrillatory waves	• Heart failure, COPD, thyrotoxicosis, constrictive pericarditis, ischemic heart disease, sepsis, pulmonary embolus, rheumatic heart disease, hypertension, mitral stenosis, atrial irritation, complication of coronary bypass or valve replacement surgery.	• If a patient is unstable with ventricular rate > 150 bpm, prepare for immediate cardioversion. • If stable drug therapy may include calcium channel blockers, beta-adrenergic blockers, digoxin, procainamide, quinidine or amiodarone. • Anticoagulation therapy to prevent emboli • Dual chamber atrial pacing implantable atrial pacemaker, or surgical maze procedure may also be used

Description	Causes	Treatment	Arrhythmias
• Atrial and ventricular rhythms are regular. • Atrial rate 40 to 60 bpm. • P waves preceding hidden within (absent) or after QRS complex; usually inverted if visible. • PR interval (when present) < 0.12 second. • QRS complex configuration and duration normal, except in aberrant conduction.	• Inferior wall MI, or ischemia, hypoxia, vagal stimulation sick sinus syndrome. • Acute rheumatic fever. • Valve surgery • Digoxin toxicity	• Correction of underlying cause. • Atropine for symptomatic slow rate. • Pacemaker insertion if patient is refractory to drugs. • Discontinuation of digoxin if appropriate.	**Junctional Rhythm** 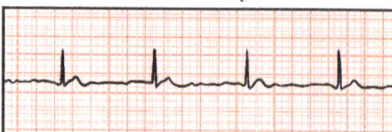

EKG INTERPRETATION RESOURCE

Arrhythmias	Description	Causes	Treatment
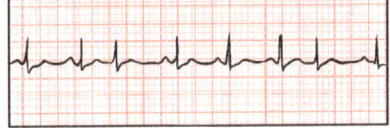 Premature Junctional Conjuctions	• Atrial and ventricular rhythms are irregular. • P waves inverted; may precede be hidden within, or follow QRS complex. • QRS complex configuration and duration normal.	• MI or ischemia. • Digoxin toxicity and excessive caffeine or amphetamine use.	• Correction of underlying cause. • Discontinuation of digoxin if appropriate.

Description	Causes	Treatment	Arrhythmias
• Atrial and ventricular rhythm regular. • PR interval> 0.20 sec • P wave preceding each QRS complex • QRS complex normal.	• Inferior wall MI or ischemia or infarction, hypothyroidism, hypokalemia, hyperkalemia • Digoxin toxicity • Use of quinidine, procainamide, beta adrenergic blocks, calcium	• Correction of the underlying cause. • Possibly atropine if PR interval exceeds 0.25 seconds or symptomatic bradycardia develops. • Cautious use of digoxin, calcium channel blockers, and beta-adrenergic blockers.	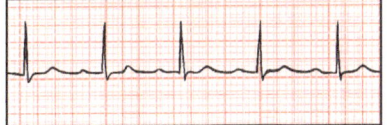 First- degree AV block

Karen Ann Thompson M.S., RN

ARTERIAL BLOOD GAS INTERPRETATION

RESPIRATORY ACIDOSIS

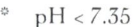

- pH < 7.35
- CO2, > 45

Causes:
COPD
Barbiturate overDOSE
Chest wall abnormality
Severe pneumothorax
Atelectasis
Gullian-Barre syndrome
Hypoventilation

Symptoms:
Rapid shallow respirations
Decreased BP w/ vasodilation
Headache
Hyperkalaemia
Dysrhythmias
Drowsiness
Disorientation
Muscle weakness and
Hyperreflexia

NORMAL BLOOD GAS LEVELS

pH 7.35-7.45: The lower the number the more acidic you are.

CO, 35-45: The greater the number the more acidic you become. CO2 is controlled by respiration.

HCO, 22-26: The lower the number the more acidic you are. Bicarb is controlled via the kidneys

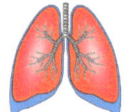

RESPIRATORY ALKALOSIS

- pH > 7.45
- CO2, < 35

Causes:
Hyperventilation
Hypoxia
PE
Septicaemia
Encephalitis
Brain injury
Salicylate poisoning
Fever
Stimulated respiratory centre.
Mechanical hyperventilation

Symptoms:
Seizures
Deep, rapid breathing.
Hyperventilation
Tachycardia
Decreased bp
Hypokalaemia
Numbness and tingling
Lethargy and confusion
Light-headedness
Nausea, vomiting

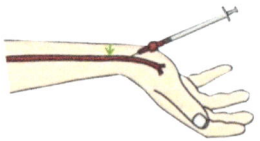

METBOLIC ACIDOSIS

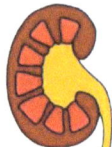

- pH < 7.35
- HCO3, < 22

Causes:
Seizures
Deep, rapid breathing.
Hyperventilation
Tachycardia
Decreased bp
Hypokalaemia
Numbness and tingling
Lethargy and confusion
Light-headedness
Nausea, vomiting

Symptoms:
Headache
Decreased Bp
Hyperkalaemia
Muscle twitching
Vasodilation (warm and flushed
Dry skin)
Nausea vomiting and diarrhoea
Contusion and drowsiness

METABOLIC ALKALOSIS

- pH > 7.45
- HCO3, > 26

Causes:
Severe vomiting
Gastric suction
Diuretic therapy
Potassium deficit
Excess NaHCO3, intake
Excess mineralocorticoids

Symptoms:
Restlessness
Lethargy
Tachycardia
Compensatory hypoventilation
Confusion
Nausea, vomiting. Diarrhoea
Tremors
Muscle cramps
Tingling in fingers/ toes

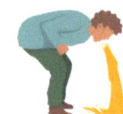

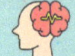

COMPENSATION
Think two chubby lids on a teeter totter, when one is up the other is down and you have to have something in normal range to achieve balance.

If pH is normal range acid/base is fully compensated.

If ph is out of range and CO2, or HCO3, are opposites then you have artial compensation.

If pH is out of range but either CO2 or HCO3, are normal then you are uncompensated.

BASIC VENTILATOR MODES & ALARMS CHEAT SHEET

	Mode	Description	Indications
Most Support ⬇	Controlled Mechanical Ventilation (CMV)	Provides *mandatory* breaths using a set rate and Vt regardless of inspiratory effort. Provides total control of the MV. • Only allows mandatory breaths from vent. Patient CANNOT trigger a breath. • Can be volume controlled (VC) or pressure controlled (PC).	• Patients who are fully sedated and paralyzed with a Neuromuscular blocking agent.
	Assist Control (A/C)	The clinician determines the tidal volume and RR (Minute Ventilation). • Breaths are either mandatory or assisted. • Breaths CAN be triggered by the patient but are delivered by the vent (i.e. an assisted breath, with a set Tv, and flow) • Can be volume controlled (VC) or pressure controlled (PC).	• Often used as an initial mode for ventilation. • Suited for the critically ill patient as it gives the most control and can take over full WOB. • Patient must be adequately sedated.
	Synchronized Intermittent Mandatory Ventilation (SIMV)	A combination mode where the clinician determines the tidal volume and RR (Minute Ventilation) but allows the patient to initiate independent breaths +/- Pressure support. • Vent support can range from full support to none. • Breaths are either mandatory, assisted, or spontaneous. • Breaths CAN be triggered by the patient (on a set pressure support) in between the set ventilator breaths (i.e. an assisted (PS) or spontaneous breath). • The mandatory ventilator breaths are synchronous to patients inspiratory efforts. • Can be volume controlled (VC) or pressure controlled (PC).	• Patients that require partial ventilation support. • Weaning mode.
	Pressure Support (PSV) *Often used with SIMV mode.*	A spontaneous breathing mode. • All breaths are patient initiated → vent delivers a pre-set positive pressure for duration of inspiration (i.e. an assisted breath) • All breaths are "assisted" by definition due to the pressure support	• Weaning mode • Long term ventilation
	Bilevel Positive Airway Pressure (BiPAP) *Non-invasive ventilation*	A spontaneous breathing mode. Every breath is supported with positive pressure. • 2 set pressures – positive inspiratory pressure (IPAP) and positive expiratory pressure (EPAP) • Must be able to spontaneously breathe and protect airway • All breaths are spontaneous	• COPD • Heart Failure • Hypoventilation • To try and avoid invasive intubation/mechanical ventilation
Least Support	Continuous Positive Airway Pressure (CPAP) *Non-invasive ventilation*	A spontaneous breathing mode. Delivers continuous pressure throughout the entire respiratory cycle. • Must be able to spontaneously breathe and protect airway • All breaths are spontaneous	• Obstructive sleep apnea • Heart Failure *Can also be used as a mode with an invasive ventilation, but not commonly seen.*

@Thenursefilesco
April 2023

Karen Ann Thompson M.S., RN

BREATH TYPES		
• **Mandatory/Controlled**- breaths initiated by vent and the vent performs all of the work of inspiration • **Assisted**- breaths initiated by patient but vent performs some of the work of inspiration • **Spontaneous** – breaths initiated by patient and patient performs all of the work of inspiration		
BREATH STRATEGIES		
Pressure Control (PC)	Delivers each breath at a constant pressure. Pressure is constant but volume varies (Vt). • Can be used in CMV, AC or SIMV. • Can be assisted or mandatory breath.	• ARDS • Stiff Lungs
Volume Control (VC)	Delivers each breath at set volume (Vt). Volume is constant but *pressure varies*. • Can be used in CMV, AC or SIMV. • Can be assisted or mandatory breath.	• Decreased LOC • Sedated • Neuromuscular dysfunction • Normal drive but weak resp muscles

BASIC VENTILATOR ALARMS. *If unable to correct quickly or patient in distress – manually ventilate with bag valve mask and call Respiratory Therapist STAT*

Alarm	Potential Causes
High Airway Pressure	• Coughing, Gagging • "Fighting" the vent, biting the tube i.e., when waking up from sedation, pain • Excessive secretions, mucus plug • Kink in tubing • Attempting to talk • Patient bearing down (i.e. having a bowel movement) • Disease such as ARDS, COPD, Large effusion, Pulmonary edema, Pneumothorax, bronchospasm etc.
Low Airway Pressure	• Disconnection of tubes • Cuff Leak • ETT displacement • Poor fitting mask • Loose circuit • Self extubation • High patient flow demand
Apnea	• Disconnection • Patient stops breathing – fatigue, over sedation, neuromuscular paralysis (i.e. need to change vent settings) • Vent failure

For Mechanically Ventilated Patients, ensure you know the following:

- Date Intubation and reason
- Size of ETT
- Vent Settings

IMPORTANT: Always refer to your facility's policy for the most reliable source of information. The information in this cheat sheet is not to be used in substitution of your institution's policies, procedures, or guidelines. This cheat sheet is a supplementary resource only.

@Thenursefilesco
April 2023

Common ICU Drips

VASOPRESSORS

MED	DESIRED EFFECT	TYPICAL STARTING DOSAGE	TITRATION AMOUNT	MAX	NOTES
Levophed (norepinephrine)	Increase BP	5 mcg/min	1-5 mcg/min, q3-5min	40 mcg/min	MUST have CVC
Vasopressin	Increase BP	0.04 units/min	No titration	NA	For sepsis; enhances Levo
Neosynephrine (Phenylophrine)	Increase BP	30 mcg/min	5-10 mcg/min q3-5min	220 mcg/min	To raise BP rapidiy. can start at 100mcg
Epinephrine	Increase BP	1-4 mcg/min	1-2 mcg/min	2-10 mcg/min is typical	Higher doses are not better; watch for increased HR
Dopamine	Increase BP	2-5 mcg/kg/min	1-4 mcg/kg/hr q10min	20 mcg/kg/min	Watch for increased HR

VASODILATORS

MED	DESIRED EFFECT	TYPICAL STARTING DOSAGE	TITRATION AMOUNT	MAX	NOTES
Cardene (Nicardipine)	Decrease BP	5 mg/hr	2.5 mg/hr q15min	15 mg/hr	Must change IV site q12hr
Esmolol	Decrease BP	25-50 mcg/kg/min	50 mcg/kg/min q4min	300 mcg/kg/min	
Nipride	Decrease BP	0.2-4mcg/kg/min	0.25-0.5 mcg/kg/Min q3-5min	10 mcg/kg/min	Can cause major hypotension

MISCELLANEOUS ICU DRIPS

MED	DESIRED EFFECT	TYPICAL STARTING DOSAGE	TITRATION AMOUNT	MAX	NOTES
Propofol (diprivan)	Sedative	10 mcg/kg/min	5 mcg/kg/min q5min	80 mcg/kg/min	Quick half life
Precedex (dexmedetomidine)	Sedative	(May qualify for loading dose) 0.2 mcg/kg/min	0.1 mcg/kg/min	1.4 mcg/kg/min (0.7 most typical)	
Cardizem	Decrease HR, Convert to NSR	5 mg/hr	5. Mg/hr q15min	20 mg/hr	
Amiodarone	Decrease HR, Convert to NSR	1mg/minx6 hours	None	NA	3 pre-mixed bags Over 24 hrs

CRITICAL CARE NURSING HEMODYNAMICS

CARDIAC OUTPUT
Amount of blood pumped by the heart in one minute. Normal cardiac output is 5.6 litters per minute

STROKE VOLUME
The volume of blood pumped out of each left ventricle of the heart during each systolic cardiac contraction

SYSTEMIC VASCULAR RESISTANCE
The resistance in the circulatory system that is used to create blood pressure, the flow of blood and is also a component of cardiac function

PRELOAD
It is the initial stretching of cardiac myocytes prior to contraction. It is related to ventricular filling (end diastolic volume).

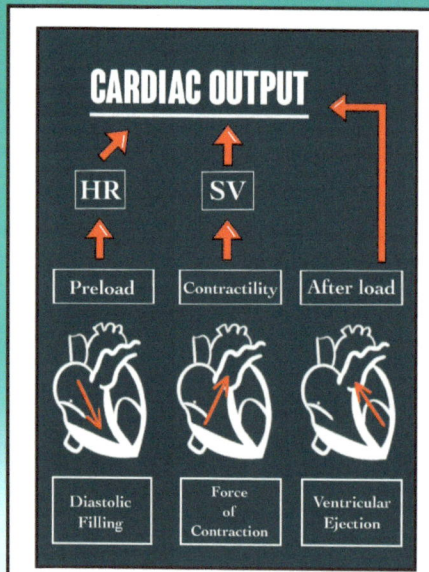

CARDIAC INDEX
An assessment of the cardiac output value based on the patients size. To find cardiac index, divide the cardiac output by the person's body surface area

STROKE VOLUME INDEX
It relates stroke volume to body surface area (BSA), thus relating heart performance to the size of the individual. Unit of measurement is ml/m2

PULMONARY VASCULAR RESISTANCE:
The resistance against blood flow from the pulmonary artery to the left atrium

AFTERLOAD
The resistance against which the heart must pump blood and is represented by aortic impedance and systemic vascular resistance

INVASIVE PRESSURE MONITORING

ARTERIAL BP

INDICATIONS:
Hemodynamic measurements (cardiac output, stroke volume), Acute pulmonary hypertension, Pulmonary embolism, Estimation of preload

MEASUREMENTS:
Carotid bp, Systolic/diastolic bp, Peripheral vascular resistance (PVR)

NURSING:
Electrocardiogram (ecg), Photoplethysmography(ppg)

VENOUS O² SATURATION:

It is the measure of oxygen content of the blood returning to the right side of the heart after perfusing the entire body.

MEASUREMENTS:
Mixed venous oxygen saturation(SvO2) and oxygen saturation(SpO2)

INTERPRETATION:
· Decreased SvO2 increased oxygen need; fever, shivering, stress, anxiety
· Decreased oxygen supply; low cardiac output, hypoxemia, anemia, hemodilution.
· Increased SvO2 Increased oxygen supply; high cardiac output, early sepsis, cyanide poisoning
Decreased oxygen need; analgesia, sedation, hypothermia

PULMONARY ARTERY FLOW-DIRECTED CATHETER

INDICATIONS: Cardiac output measurement, unequal right and left ventricular failure, complex hemodynamic stability, to differentiate cardiogenic pulmonary edema from non cardiogenic

MEASUREMENTS: Pulmonary artery catheter simultaneously measures pressures in the right atrium, right ventricle, pulmonary artery and the filling pressure.

ARTERIAL PRESSURE-BASED CARDIAR OUTPUT (APCO)

INDICATIONS:
Measures the rate of flow (cardiac output). Stroke volume and heart rate are key determinants of cardiac output.

MEASUREMENTS:
Use an arterial catheter. Mean arterial pressure(MAP), stroke volume, cardiac output

CONTRAINDICATIONS:
Absent pulse, raynaud syndrome, thickness of skin due to burns intra aortic balloon pump therapy (IABP)

CENTRAL VENOUS PRESSURE:

MEASUREMENTS:
CVP is the pressure recorded from the right atrium pr superior vena cava and is representative of the filling pressure of the right side of heart

INTERPRETATION:
Raised CVP : Right ventricular failure, tricuspid stenosis, superior vena caval obstruction, fluid overload.

Decreased CVP :
Fall in effective circulating volume, venodilation.

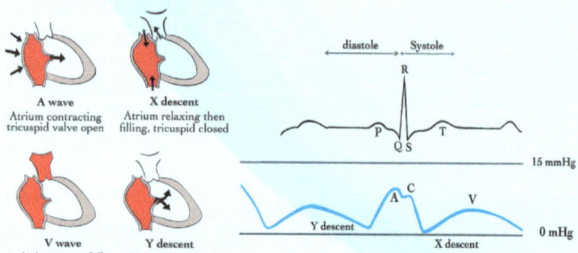

Deep Tendon Reflexes

4+ very brisk, hyperactive

3+ brisker than average, slightly hyperactive

0 absent

2+ average, normal

1+ somewhat diminished, below average

Glasgow Coma Scale

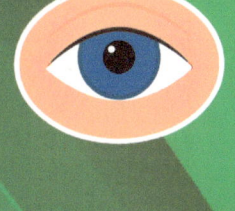

SPONTANEOUS	4
TO SOUND	3
TO PRESSURE	2
NONE	1

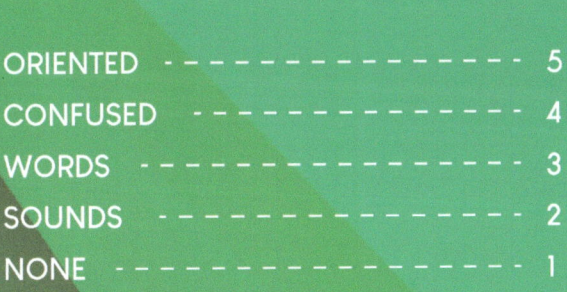

ORIENTED	5
CONFUSED	4
WORDS	3
SOUNDS	2
NONE	1

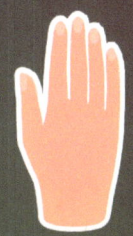

OBEY COMMANDS	6
LOGALIZING	5
NORMAL FIEXION	4
ABNORMAL FLEXION	3
EXTENSION	2
NONE	1

LESS THAN 8 = INTUBATE

Karen Ann Thompson M.S., RN

EKG Interpretation Resource

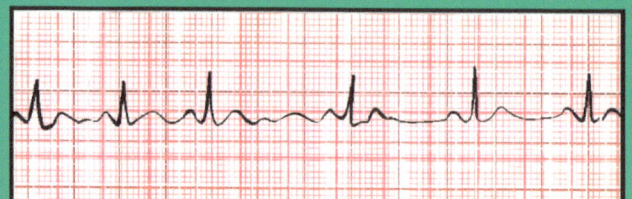

Arrhythmias — **Sinus Arrhythmia**

Description
- Irregular atrial and ventricular rhythms.
- Normal P wave preceding each QRS complex

Causes
- Normal variation of sinus rhythm in athletes, children, and the elderly.
- Can be seen in digoxin toxicity and inferior wall MI.i

Treatment
- Atropine if rate decreases below 40bpm.

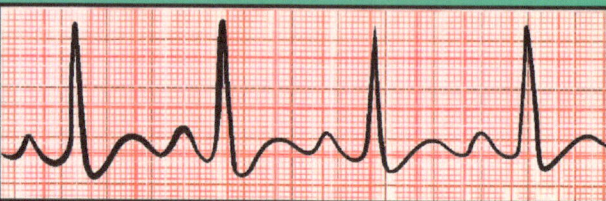

Arrhythmias — **Sinus Tachycardia**

Description
- Atrial and ventricular rhythms are regular.
- Rate > 100 bpm
- Normal P wave preceding each QRS complex.

Causes
- Normal physiologic response to fever exercise. anxiety. dehydration or pain.
- May accompany shock, left-sided Beta-adrenergic heart failure, cardiac tamponade, hyperthyroidism and anemia.
- Atropine, epinephrine, quinidine, carteine, nicotine and alcohol use.

Treatment
- Correction of underlying cause.
- Atropine, epinephrine, quinidine, carteine, nicotine and alcohol use.

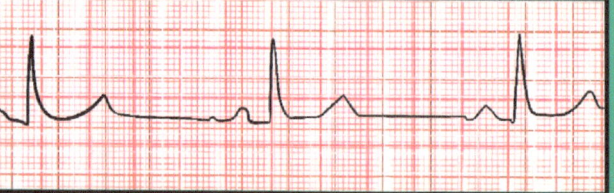

Arrhythmias — **Sinus Bradycardia**

Description
- Regular atrial and ventricular rhythms.
- Rate < 60 bpm
- Normal P wave preceding each QRS complex.

Causes
- Normal in a well-conditioned heart (e.g athletes)
- Increased intracranial pressure;
- Increased vagal tone due to straining during defecation, vomiting, incubation, mechanical ventilation.

Treatment
- Follow ACLS protocol for administration of atropine for symptoms of low cardiac output, dizziness, weakness, altered LOC, or low blood pressure.
- Pacemaker

EKG Interpretation Resource

Arrhythmias

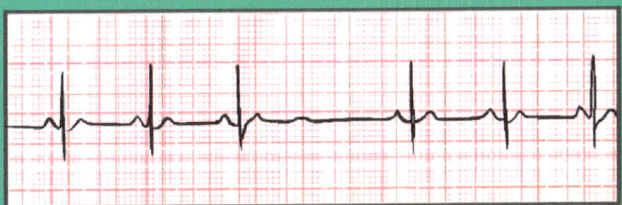

Sinoatrial (SA) arrest or block

Description
- Atrial and ventricular rhythms are normal except for missing complexes.
- Normal P wave preceding each QRS complex.
- Pause not equal to multiple for the previous rhythm.

Causes
- Infection.
- Coronary artery disease, degenerative heart disease, acute inferior wall MI.
- Vagal stimulation, Valsalva maneuver, carotid sinus massage.

Treatment
- Treat symptoms with atropine I.V.
- Temporary pacemaker or permanent pacemaker if considered for repeated episodes.

Arrhythmias

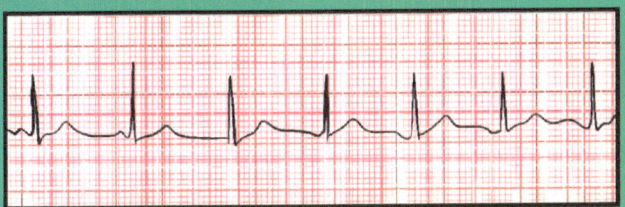

Wandering atrial pacemaker

Description
- Atrial and ventricular rhythms vary slightly.
- Irregular PR interval.
- P waves irregular with changing configuration indicating that they aren't all from SA node or single atrial focus may appear after the QRS complex.
- QRS complexes are uniform in shape but irregular in rhythm.

Causes
- Rheumatic carditis due to inflammation involving the SA node.
- Digoxin toxicity.
- Sick sinus syndrome.

Treatment
- No treatment if patient is asymptomatic.
- Treatment of underlying cause if patient is symptomatic.

Arrhythmias

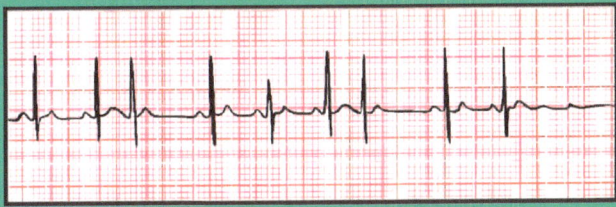

Premature atrial contraction (PAC)

Description
- Premature, abnormal looking P waves that differ in configuration from normal P waves.
- QRS complexes after P waves except in very early or blocked PACs.
- P wave often buried in the preceding T wave.

Causes
- May prelude supraventricular tachycardia.
- Stimulants, hyperthyroidism, COPD, infection and other heart diseases.

Treatment
- Usually no treatment is needed.
- Treatment of underlying causes if the patient is symptomatic.
- Carotid sinus massage

HEMODYNAMIC PARAMETERS

CARDIAC INDEX (CI)

Cardiac output per body surface area

Normal: 2.5 - 4.0 L/min/m

CARDIAC OUTPUT (CO)

Total volume of blood pumped by the heart per min

Normal: 4 - 8 L/min

CENTRAL VENOUS PRESSURE (CVP)

Measure of pressure in the superior vena cava

Normal: 2 - 8 mmHg

MEAN ARTERIAL PRESSURE (MAP)

Average arterial pressure throughout one cardiac cycle - systole and diastole

Normal: 70 - 100 mmHg
Must be at least 60 mmHg for adequate perfusion of vital organs

SYSTEMIC VASCULAR RESISTANCE (SVR)

The resistance exerted on circulating blood by the vasculature of the body.

Normal: 800 - 1200 dynes/sec/cm

ICU RESOURCE SHEET

ABGs	pH	pCO2	HCO3	Common causes
Normal	7.35-7.45	35-45	22-26	
Respiratory Acidosis	↓	↑	Normal or ↑	Respiratory depression (Drugs, CNS trauma) COPD
Respiratory Alkalosis	↑	↓	Normal or ↓	Hyperventilation (Anxiety, Pain)
Metabolic Acidosis	↓	Normal or ↓	↓	Diabetes, Shock, Renal failure
Metabolic Alkalosis	↑	Normal or ↑	↑	Sodium Bicarbonate oxidation, Prolonged vomiting, NG drainage

Alpha 1	Vasoconstriction
Alpha 2	CNS, Decreases sympathetic outflow
Beta 1	Cardiac cells, Increased heart rate, Increased contractility, Increased renin release
Beta 2	Relaxes smooth muscle, Relax Bronchi

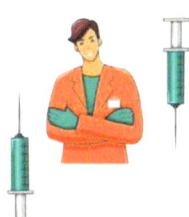

ELECTROLYTE LAB	NORMAL VALUE	S/S OF ABNORMALITY
Sodium	135-145	↑ALOC, Restlessness, Agitation ↓cerebral edema, nausea, seizures
Potassium	3.5-5	↑Muscle weakness, arrhythmias, peaked T waves, wide QRS complex ↓Muscle weakness, cramps, rhabdomyolysis
Magnesium	2-3	C↑↓Deep tendon reflex, ↓BP,↓HR, muscle paralysis ↓Tetany, Arrhythmias(Torsade de pointes)
Calcium	8-10	↑Polyuria, Polydipsia, muscle weakness ↓Tetany
Phosphorous	2.5-4.5	↑Effects of ↓Ca, ↓Effects of ↑Ca (Phosphorous and calcium are inversely proportional)
Ammonia	0-55	↑Encephalopathy

-GCS-

Eye opening Response	Spontaneously	4
	To speech	3
	To pain	2
	No response	1
Verbal Response	Oriented x3	5
	Confused	4
	Inappropriate words	3
	Incomprehensible sounds	2
	No response	1
Motor Response	Obeys commands	6
	Moves to localized pain	5
	Withdraw from pain	4
	Abnormal flexion	3
	Abnormal extension	2
	No response	1

COMMON VENTILATOR MOODS

MODE	DESCRIPTION	SPECIAL ROUTES
Continuous mandatory Ventilation(CMV)	Set tidal volume delivered at a set respiratory rate. Patient is unable to trigger breaths.	Used for paralyzed or sedated patients.
Synchronized intermittent mandatory ventilation(SIMV)	Mandatory breaths synchronized with spontaneous breaths. Patient triggered breaths given at tidal volume generated by patient.	Can decrease cardiac output in patients with left ventricular dysfunction
Pressure controlled ventilation (PCV)	Ventilator initiated breaths set to a predetermined pressure level. Tidal volumes vary in order to achieve set pressure	Used for patients with neuromuscular disease. Patients do not trigger breaths
Pressure support ventilation (PSV)	Patient triggers respiratory frequency and inflation volume. Ventilator controls pressure.	Used to augment spontaneous breathing
Airway pressure release ventilation (APRV)	Positive airway pressure augments spontaneous inspiration. Pressure level is reduced to allow for exhalation	Decreases incidence of barotrauma. No set rate. Good for patients with obstructive lung disease.

LUNG SOUNDS

RATES/CRACKLES	Bubbling or popping sound. Caused by increase fluid in the alveoli
Ronchi	A continous, low-pitched sound that can be heard on inspiration and expiration. Usually caused by secretions or blockages in the upper airway
Wheezing	High pitched musical sound that can be heard on inspiration and/or expiration. Caused by air flowing through constricted airways.
Stridor	A special kind of wheeze. A loud musical sound heard in patients with tracheal or laryngeal obstruction. Place stethoscope over the trachea rather than over the lungs.

V/Q RATIO	0.8 L/min
P2O2	80-100%
S2O2 (% of oxygen dissolved in plasma)	92-99%
P2O2/(F)O2 RATIO	300-500mmHg
PA PRESSURE	10-20 mmHg
TIDAL VOLUME	6-5ml/kg
CARDIAC OUTPUT	5 L/min

TEMPERATURE	>100.4 F / <96.8 F
HR	>90
RR	>20
WBC	>12,000 / <4,000 / >10% bands
PCO2	<32 mmHg

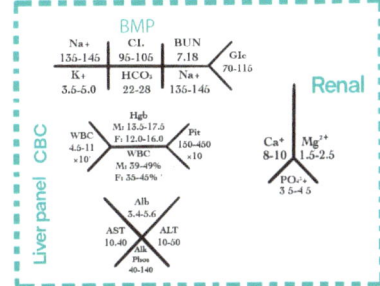

Karen Ann Thompson M.S., RN

ICU NURSING ABBREVIATIONS

BASICS

- **Rx** Pharmacy
- **Dx** Diagnosis
- **Hx** History
- **Sx** Symptoms
- **Fx** Fracture
- **Tx** Treatment
- **Ax** Allergies
- **H&P** History & Physical

- **FC** Full Code
- **DNR** Do Not Resuscitate
- **DNI** Do Not Intubate
- **DNRA** DNR- Active Tx
- **POA** Power or Attorney
- **NKA** No Known Allergies
- **NKDA** No Known Drug Allergies
- **ACLS** Advanced Care Life Support
- **BLS** Basic Life Support
- **PALS** Paediatric Advanced Life Support
- **CPR** Cardiopulmonary Resuscitation
- **ROSC** Return of Spontaneous Circulation
- **LLE** Left Lower Extremity
- **RLE** Right Lower Extremity
- **RUE** Right Upper Extremity
- **LUE** Left Upper Extremity
- **HEENT** Head, Ears, Eyes, Nose, Throat

Neuro

- **CX1-12** Cranial Nerves 1-12
- **A&0x3** Alert and Oriented x 3
- **CNS** Central Nervous System
- **PNS** Peripheral Nervous System
- **CVA** Cerebrovascular Accident
- **TIA** Transient Ischemic Attack
- **TPA** Tissue Plasminogen Activator
- **LKW** Last Known Well
- **LOC** Loss of Consciousness
- **FC** Follow: Command:
- **MAE** Moves All Extremities
- **PERRLA** Pupils Equal Round & Reactive
- **NIH** Stroke Scale Score
- **LP** Lumbar Puncture
- **CEA** Carotid Endarterectomy

Surgery

- **POD#** Post-Op Day #
- **EBL.** Estimated Blood Loas
- **PRBC** Packed Red Blood Cell:
- **Hgb** Haemoglobin
- **Hct** Haematocrit
- **H&H** Hgb & Hct
- **PT** Physical Therapy
- **OT** Occupational Therapy
- **ROM** Range of Motion
- **PCA** Patient-controlled Analgesic

Lines & Drips

- **Gtt** Drip
- **IV** Intravenous
- **CVC** Central Venous Catheter
- **IO** Intraosseous
- **IVPB** IV Piggyback
- **KVO** Keep Vein Open
- **NS** Normal Saline

GI

- **N&V** Nouse & Vomiting
- **TPN** Total Parenteral Nutrition
- **TF** Tube Feeding
- **OGT** Orogastric Tube
- **NGT** Nasogastric Tube
- **FF** Flexi-Flow
- **DHT** Dobhoff Tube
- **BMS/FMS** Bowel/Faecal Management System
- **Peg** Percutaneous Endoscopic Gastrostomy
- **JP** Jackson-Pratt
- **OMI** Type 1 Diabetes
- **DMII** Type 2 Diabetes
- **ACHS** Before Meal & at Bedtime
- **ExLap** Exploratory Laparotomy

Skin & Activity

- **PU** Pressure Ulcer
- **PUI-4** Pressure Ulcer Stage 1 to 4
- **Total Assist** Incapable of participating in care
- **X1 Assist** 1 person assist to stand
- **X2 Assist** 2 person assist to stand
- **Ad Lib** As desired activity

Types of SHOCK

Though all labs are generally affected by SHOCK this critical thinking evaluation of the causes are in monitoring all labs for on going evaluation of treatment and complications

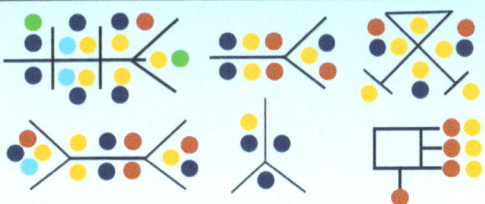

COMMON LABS IN SHOCK

Lactic Aid - <4	Osmolality 280-300
Anion Gap - 5 -15	U-Osmolality 38-1400
Troponin-I 0.0-0.1	Urine Na —60-260
Troponin -T >0.4	PH 7.35-7.45
CPK- <150	PCO2-35-45
CPK-MB <50	HCO3– 22-26
Fibrinogen — 145-450	SVO2– 60-80 %
Plasminogen 60-120%	PaO2– 80-100 %
D-Dimer <250	U- Spec Grav 1.001-1.035

Lab & Organ AFFECTED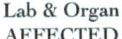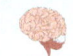

Type	Anaphylactic	Cardiogenic	Hypovolemic	Neurogenic	Septic
	Allergic	Pump Failure	Low Volume	Neuro Shock	Septicemia
BP/MAP >70 mmHg	v	v	v	v	v
CO-4-8 LPM	^	v	v	^	^
HR-60-100	^	^v	^	v	^
SV-60-120	–	v	v	–	v^
SVR-700-1200 -Resistance	v	^	^	v	v
EF- >60 — Percent output	–	v	^	–	v
Skin Temperature	v	v	v	^v	^v
JVD <4 (right sided Volume)	^	^	v	v	v
CVP 2-8 (Right sided Volume)	^	^	v	v	v
PAWP 8-12 (left Atrial Volume)	^	^	v	v	v
Possible Medications	Epinephrine, corticosteroids	Lasix, Dobutamine Nitroprusside	IV Fluid Bolus, blood-Underlying	IVF, Atropine, Vasopressors	Dobutamine, IV, ABX, levophed
Medical Treatments	May Intubate	Foley, TCL, PUMP	NS, O2, TX Cause	Protect Spine	SEPSIS BUNDLE

Vasopressors and Inotropic Medications used for Shock-Always Assess Fluid Status Prior to Medications

α- Alpha Agonist-(AWAY) Causing vasoconstriction β-Beta Agonist- (Beat the heart) Causing beta cells on heart to pump

Medication for shock	SVR	MAP	HR	CO
Dopamine αβ=Beta low doses>10α 0.5-20mcg/kg/min	^	^	^	^
Milrinone 0.375-0.75 mcg/kg/min	v	v	–	^
Nitroprusside 3-10 mcg/kg/minute	v	v	^	^

Medication for shock	SVR	MAP	HR	CO
Phenylephrine - α1 20-300mcg/min	^	^	v	v
Vasopressin V1 0.01-0.1 u/min	^	^	v	v
Norepinephrine α1 greater than β1 5-0 mcg/min	^	^	^	^
Epinephrine α1 α2 β1 β2 2-30 mcg/min	v^	^	^	^
Isoproterenol 1β2 0.1-10 mcg/min	v	v	^	^
Dobutamine= β1 > β2 2-20 mcg/kg/min	v	v	^	^

Karen Ann Thompson M.S., RN

ICU SHIFT REPORT

NAME:	BED:	AGE:	M/F

Admit Date/Diagnosis:

Course in hospital:

Past Medical Hx:

Past Surgical Hx:

ALERTS | PROVIDERS | SOCIAL

Code Status:
Airway:
Allergies:
Isolation:
Safety:
Falls:

MRP:

Consults:

From:

SDM:

NEURO | RESP

LOC: Orientation: GCS:
Pupils: Speech:
Motor Strength Upper (L/R):
Motor Strength Lower (L/R):

☐ Sedation: Awakening trials:
RASS Current: Goal:
☐ Paralytic: Trainof4:

☐ Restraints:

☐ Delirium:

☐ ICP: EVD:

Pain: Analgesic: Last dose:

O2:   FiO2:   RR:
NP/ NRB / HF / BIPAP / CPAP / VENT
SpO2:   SvO2:

☐ Trach: Size & Type:
☐ Cuff Up / Down / Corked
Lung Sounds: Cough:
Secretions:

VENT

Date Intubation: Date Extubation:

ETT Size: Length: @ lip / teeth
Vent mode: Rate:
P/S: FiO2:
Vt: Peep: Peak:
Spont trial:

ABG:

CARDIAC | ACCESS/INFUSIONS

Rhythm: Dysrythmias:
HR: PR: Temp:
Pulses: Heart sounds:
CSMW:
EF%:   Edema:

☐ A-line: BP A-line: BP Cuff:
Current MAP: GOAL MAP:
CVP: CO:
CI: SVR:

Pacemaker:
☐ PPM: _____
☐ TPM: TCP / TVP- Access site:
  TPM Pacer Settings:
    Mode: Rate: mA: mV:

ACCESS TYPE	FLUID/MED	RATE

ICU SHIFT REPORT

GI		GU	
Abd:	N/V:	Continent / Incontinent	
Blood glucose:		☐ Catheter Size:	Date inserted:
Insulin: SubQ / Infusion			
Diet:	Fluid Restrict:	☐ CRRT / HD / PD	Frequency:
☐ OG/ NG/ NJ / PEG @ _____ cm		**FLUID BALANCE**	
☐ Suction:		Shift ins:	
☐ Feeds:			
Current Rate:	Goal Rate:	Shift out:	Cumulative:
Flushes:	Suction:		
Last BM:	Rectal Tube:		

SKIN/WOUNDS/INCISIONS/DRAINS	MSK/ACTIVITY	DIAGNOSTICS
Skin: Wound/Incisions: _____ _____ _____ _____ _____ Drains/tubes:	Activity: Mobility / Assist Device: Turns: VTE prophylaxis:	Last CXR:

LABS				MICROBIOLOGY	MEDS
Na:	Cl:	BUN:	Gluc:	Cultures:	
K:	HCO3:	Cr:	GFR:	Active Infection/site:	
Ca:	Mg:	Phos:			
WBC:	Hgb:	HCT:	Plts:	Antibiotics:	
INR:	PTT:	PT:			
Lactate:	Trop:	BNP:			

SHIFT TO DO LIST		CURRENT ISSUES & PATIENT PLAN	
0700	1400	ISSUES:	PLAN:
0800	1500		
0900	1600		
1000	1700	ROUNDS/NEW ORDERS:	SHIFT UPDATES:
1100	1800		
1200	1900		
1300	2000		

Oxygen Delivery Devices Cheat Sheet

> Room air = 21 % FiO2
> 1L = FiO2 approximately 24 % *(FiO2 concentration increases by ~ 3-4% for every L of oxygen)*
> **Reminder oxygen is high combustible! No smoking or flammable material **

Low Flow System *Delivers a flowrate that is below a patients inspiratory flow demand, does not deliver a precise FiO2*			
	Flow	FiO2 %	Notes
Nasal Prongs or Cannula	1-6 LPM	~ 24-44%	- Comfortable and usually well tolerated - Used for mild hypoxia, basic oxygen needs - Can be used for short or long term use - Humidity recommended if >4L - Monitor for skin breakdown at nares and back of ears - May not be a good device for mouth breathers
Simple Face Mask	6-10 LPM	~40-60%	- Used for short term stabilization of desaturating patient - *Minimum 6L flow required* for CO2 clearance - Consider using for mouth breathers - Often used after extubation from surgical procedure - Patient is unable to eat or drink while wearing - Monitor for skin breakdown at bridge of nose and back of ears - Not used long term
Non-Rebreather (NRB)	10-15 LPM	~up to 95%	- Used in emergency desaturation situations - Ensure reservoir bag is inflated before applying to patient face. If reservoir bag fully deflates on inspiration (increase oxygen flow) as it should only partially deflate. - Patient is unable to eat or drink while wearing - A health care provider should be at the bedside at all times. If the patient is left unattended one of the one way valves needs to be removed to prevent accidental suffocation if oxygen runs out or tubing kinks. - Short term use only → can lead to oxygen toxicity. If high amounts of oxygen are needed for a prolong time RT should set up a high flow system - Also used during carbon monoxide poising
Bag Valve Mask (Ambubag)	15 LPM	100%	- Resuscitation device - Delivers breaths to patient when user squeezes the bag - Can be used with face mask or can detach the face mask and attach to endotracheal tube (ET) if patient is intubated

@Thenursefilesco
2022

Oxygen Delivery Devices Cheat Sheet

High Flow System			
Delivers a flowrate that meets or exceeds their inspiratory flow demand, delivers a precise FiO2			
	Flow	FiO2	Notes
Venturi Mask	2-15 LPM	24-60%	<ul><li>For patients that require a fixed amount of oxygen</li><li>For patients with chronic hypercarbia with moderate hypoxemia (i.e. COPD)</li><li>Color coded adapter administers precise oxygen concentration:</li><li>BLUE = 2-4L/min = 24% O2</li><li>WHITE = 4-6L/min = 28% O2</li><li>YELLOW = 8-10L/min = 35% O2</li><li>RED = 10-12L/min = 40% O2</li><li>GREEN = 12-15L/min = 60% O2</li><li>Patient is unable to eat, drink or talk while wearing</li></ul>
High Flow Nasal Cannula (i.e. Opti flow)	30-60 LPM	21-100%	<ul><li>Heated humidity</li><li>Specific FiO2 is set (usually only RTs can adjust this)</li><li>Good choice if patient requires high oxygen levels but doesn't need ventilation support</li></ul>
Face Tent	10-15 LPM	~40%	Used for:<ul><li>Those who feel claustrophobic or don't tolerate the face mask</li><li>Those with facial burns or trauma</li></ul>

Trach masks are also considered high flow and require humidification.

Please note there is variation among textbooks regarding FiO2 numbers of different devices – refer to your hospital manufacturer.

IMPORTANT: Always refer to your facility's policy for the most reliable source of information. The information in this cheat sheet is not to be used in substitution of your institution's policies, procedures, or guidelines. This cheat sheet is a supplementary resource only

@Thenursefilesco
2022

Vasopressors and Inotropes

Alpha I: affects arteries, ↑vascular tone, ↑BP (ex: Phenylephrine)
Beta I: heart stimulation, ↑HR, ↑contractility, ↑arrhythmias (ex: Dopamine)

Neosynephrine = Alpha I agonist
- Powerful drug! Used when no beta stimulation is wanted or needed
- Causes vasoconstriction, bradycardia
- ↑BP, ↑SVR, ↑PVR, ↑afterload
- Coronary vasoconstriction
- May need to add dopamine to keep HR up
- Used a lot in neuro d/t the disruption of alpha system in neuro shock
- Dosing: start at 100-180 mcg/min, then 40-60
- Titrate: 5mcg q 15-minutes

Dopamine = Beta I & Alpha I agonist
- First line agent for many shock states
- Naturally-occurring catecholamine
- Precursor to norepinephrine
- 1-3 mcg/kg/min → renal, coronary, cerebral vasodilation (not renal protective!) ↑UO
- 3-10 mcg/kg/min → Beta I stimulation with positive inotropic effect, ↑HR, ↑BP
- >10 mcg/kg/min → Alpha I stimulation with potent vasoconstriction, ↑BP, ↑SVR

Norepinephrine = Alpha 1 & 2 agonist
- Endogenous catecholamine; has powerful inotrophic and peripheral vasoconstriction effects
- Arterial and venous constriction
- ↑BP, HR may slow, CO unchanged or ↓d/t increased afterload
- ↑SVR and PVR
- Dosing: 2-10 mcg/min

Epinephrine = Beta I & Alpha I agonist
- Endogenous catecholamine
- POWERFUL inotropic, peripheral and global vasoconstriction
- Not first line treatment...too potent!
- ↑contractility and ↑heart O2 demands
- ↑HR, ↑MAP, ↑CO, ↑SVR and PVR
- Causes arrhythmias :-(
- Dosing: 1-4 mcg/min

Dobutamine = Beta I agonist
- A synthetic catecholamine
- Used for + inotropic properties when vasoconstriction undesirable, reduces preload and afterload
- Commonly used with another catecholamine or vasodilator
- ↑contractility, ↑CO, ↑BP, ↑myocardial O2 demands, ↑HR
- If pt is dry, it may drop the BP
- Dosing: 2.5 - 20 mcg/kg/min
- Titrate: 1-2 mcg/kg/min q 5-10 min

Vasopressin = Vasopressin I agonist
- Anti-diuretic hormone
- Used in ACLS for pulseless VT and VF
- Smooth muscle constriction (including bronchioles)
- Less constriction at coronary and renal beds
- Vasodilates cerebral vasculature
- May enhance platelet aggregation in septic shock
- ↑BP, ↑MAP, ↑SVR, ↓UO
- Dosing usually .03 or .04 units/min

Milrinone = PDE inhibitor
- Positive inotrope and vasodilator
- Cleared by the liver
- Increases cAMP → more Ca into cells → improves myocardial contractility while inhibiting vasoconstriction.
- ↑CO, ↓CVP, ↓SVR
- Loading dose: 50 mcg/kg over 10 min
- Maintenance dose: 0.375-0.75 mcg/kg/min

❋ **Milrinone can ONLY be mixed with NS!**

Resources

Abbasinia, Mohammad, Fazlollah Ahmadi, and Anoshirvan Kazemnejad. 2019. "Patient Advocacy in Nursing: A Concept Analysis." *Nursing Ethics*, 27 (1): 141–151. https://doi.org/10.1177/0969733019832950

Aghaie, Bahman, Reza Norouzadeh, Ehsan Sharifipour, Alireza Koohpaei, Reza Negarandeh, and Mohammad Abbasinia. 2021. "The Experiences of Intensive Care Nurses in Advocacy of COVID-19 Patients." *Journal of Patient Experience*, 8. https://doi.org/10.1177/23743735211056534

Agency for Healthcare Research and Quality, "TeamSTEPPS®." Accessed July 19, 2022. https://www.ahrq.gov/teamstepps/instructor/scenarios/icu.html#scene48

Allnurses, 2017. "ICU Certifications?" allnurses.com, January 9, 2017. https://allnurses.com/icu-certifications-t635154/

Arshad, Muhammad, Neelam Qasim, Omer Farooq, and John Rice. 2021. "Empowering Leadership and Employees' Work Engagement: A Social Identity Theory Perspective." *Management Decision*, 60 (5): 1218–1236. https://doi.org/10.1108/md-11-2020-1485

Bal, Daniel. 2023. "How to Become a Critical Care Nurse." *NurseJournal*, April 12, 2023. https://nursejournal.org/careers/critical-care-nurse/how-to-become/

Brosche, Theresa Ann. 2003. "Death, Dying, and the ICU Nurse." *Dimensions of Critical Care Nursing*, 22 (4): 173–179. https://doi.org/10.1097/00003465-200307000-00006

Chang, Sin Mun, Pawan Budhwar, and Jonathan Crawshaw. 2021. "The Emergence of Value-Based Leadership Behavior at the Frontline of Management: A Role Theory Perspective and Future Research Agenda." *Frontiers in Psychology*, 12. https://doi.org/10.3389/fpsyg.2021.635106

Cook, Deborah, and Graeme Rocker. 2014. "Dying with Dignity in the Intensive Care Unit." *New England Journal of Medicine*, 370 (26): 2506–2514. https://doi.org/10.1056/nejmra1208795

Cottrell, Damon, and Stephanie M. Kendall. 2010. "Are You Ready to Move into Critical Care?" *Nursing*, 40 (1): 20–21. https://doi.org/10.1097/01.nurse.0000387064.52873.08

Enticott, Joanne, Sandra Braaf, Alison Johnson, Angela Jones, and Helena J. Teede. 2020. "Leaders' Perspectives on Learning Health Systems: A Qualitative Study." *BMC Health Services Research*, 20 (1). https://doi.org/10.1186/s12913-020-05924-w

Faubion, Darby. n.d. "12 Ways to Show Compassion in Nursing (With Examples)." *nursingprocess.org*. https://www.nursingprocess.org/compassion-in-nursing.html

Hayes, Margaret M., Souvik Chatterjee, and Richard M. Schwartzstein. 2017. "Critical Thinking in Critical Care: Five Strategies to Improve Teaching and Learning in the Intensive Care Unit." *Annals of the American Thoracic Society*, 14 (4): 569–575. https://doi.org/10.1513/AnnalsATS.201612-1009AS

Herrity, Jennifer. 2023. "5 Top Critical Thinking Skills (And How to Improve Them)." *indeed.com*. Last modified February 24, 2023. https://www.indeed.com/career-advice/career-development/critical-thinking-skills

Indeed Editorial Team. 2022a. "Advocacy Strategies in Nursing: Definition, Benefits and How-To." *indeed.com*. Last modified June 24, 2022. https://www.indeed.com/career-advice/career-development/advocacy-strategies-in-nursing

———. 2022b. "ICU Nursing Skills: Definition and Examples." *indeed.com*. Last modified June 24, 2022. https://www.indeed.com/career-advice/resumes-cover-letters/icu-nursing-skills

Mercadante, Sebastiano, Cesare Gregoretti, and Andrea Cortegiani. 2018. "Palliative Care in Intensive Care Units: Why, Where, What, Who, When, How." *BMC Anesthesiology*, 18 (106). https://doi.org/10.1186/s12871-018-0574-9

Morris, Gayle. 2023. "The Value of Critical Thinking in Nursing." *NurseJournal.org*, March 16, 2023. https://nursejournal.org/articles/the-value-of-critical-thinking-in-nursing/

Nurse Break Team. 2019. "Amazing Cheat Sheet Guide for Our ICU Nursing Placement." thenursebreak.org, May 9, 2019. https://thenursebreak.org/icu-nursing-placement/

NurseZone Writing Staff, 2019. "ICU Nurse Certifications: What Are They and Do You Need Them?" *americanmobile.com*, June 20, 2019. https://www.americanmobile.com/nursezone/career-development/icu-nurse-certifications-what-are-they-and-do-you-need-them/

Project Heartbeat. 2021 "5 Tips for Moving from General Floor to Critical Care Nursing." https://projectheartbeat.com/from-general-floor-to-critical-care-nursing/

Serafin, Lena, Natalia Pawlak, Zuzanna Strząska-Kliś, Anna Bobrowska, and Bożena Czarkowska-Pączek. 2021. "Novice Nurses' Readiness to Practice in an ICU: A Qualitative Study." *Nursing in Critical Care*, 27 (1): 10–18. https://doi.org/10.1111/nicc.12603

Short, Kathleen, Kara Freedman, Jennie Matays, Melody Rosamilia, and Kara Wade. 2019. "Making the Transition." *Clinical Nurse Specialist*, 33 (3): 123–127. https://doi.org/10.1097/nur.0000000000000444

Smith, Carlton R. 2014. "True Suffering in an ICU." *RN Journal*. https://rn-journal.com/journal-of-nursing/true-suffering-in-an-intensive-care-unit-icu

Stewart, Carolyne. 2021. "Understanding New Nurses' Learning Experiences in Intensive Care." *Intensive and Critical Care Nursing*, 67. https://doi.org/10.1016/j.iccn.2021.103094

Su, Amanda, Lindsay Lief, David Berlin, Zara Cooper, Daniel Ouyang, John Holmes, Renee Maciejewski, Paul K. Maciejewski, and Holly G. Prigerson. 2018. "Beyond Pain: Nurses' Assessment of Patient Suffering, Dignity, and Dying in the Intensive Care Unit." *Journal of Pain and Symptom Management*, 55 (6): 1591–1598.e1. https://doi.org/10.1016/j.jpainsymman.2018.02.005

Tang, Charmaine Jinxiu, Yongxing Patrick Lin, and Ee-Yuee Chan. 2021. "'From Expert to Novice', Perceptions of General Ward Nurses on Deployment to Outbreak Intensive Care Units During the Covid-19 Pandemic: A Qualitative Descriptive Study." *Journal of Clinical Nursing*. https://doi.org/10.1111/jocn.16029

Welch, Teresa D., and Melondie Carter. 2020. "Expertise Among Critical Care Nurses: A Grounded Theory Study." *Intensive and Critical Care Nursing*, 57. https://doi.org/10.1016/j.iccn.2019.102796

Yoo, Hye Jin, Oak Bun Lim, and Jae Lan Shim. 2020. "Critical Care Nurses' Communication Experiences with Patients and Families in an Intensive Care Unit: A Qualitative Study." *PLOS One*, 15 (7). https://doi.org/10.1371/journal.pone.0235694

Notes

www.ingramcontent.com/pod-product-compliance
Ingram Content Group UK Ltd.
Pitfield, Milton Keynes, MK11 3LW, UK
UKHW060833270426

12049UKWH00036B/163